The Chocolate Diet (and why it works)

By

Lynne D M Noble

Copyright 2020 Lynne D M Noble

This book shall not, by way of trade or otherwise, be lent, re-sold, hired out, or otherwise circulated without the prior consent of the copyright holder or the publisher in any form of binding or cover than that in which it is published and without a similar condition including this condition being imposed on the subsequent purchaser.

The use of its contents in another media is also subject to the same conditions.

Independently published

Contents

Dedication

To Rob Williams

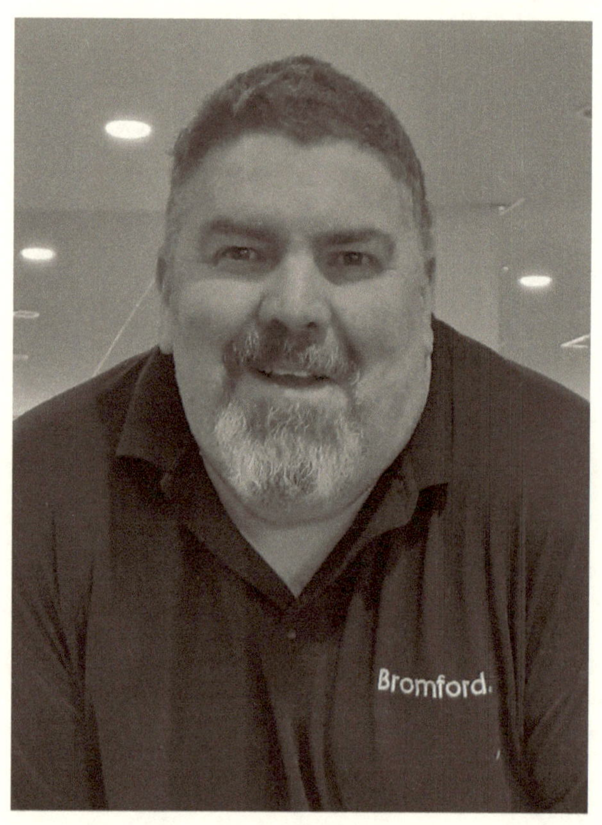

Thanks for taking an interest in my work

About the Author

Lynne Noble was born in 1953 in Huddersfield, West Yorkshire. From a very early age, Lynne showed an interest in nutrition and genetics avidly reading any books that she could get her hands on at the time.

Initially, Lynne studied orthopaedics but events led her to work with the elderly mentally infirm. Here, her interest in neurodegenerative disorders and pain syndromes developed.

Lynne undertook rigorous programmes of study, completing her Cert Ed., (FE) BSc (Hons) and Adv. Dip Education simultaneously before moving onto her M.Ed.

From there she took further demanding programmes in Human Nutrition, Pharmacology, Neuroscience, Genetics and Immunology. During this time, she was given many prestigious awards for her academic work. It was noted then that Lynne was not afraid of tackling difficult subjects.

She began her law degree but ill health prevented her from pursuing this. However, in this time, she moved from being a foster parent to adoptive parent.

She has been instrumental in setting up projects in the community for disadvantaged groups.

She is a member of the Guild of Health Writers.

Now retired, she lives in a picturesque village in West Yorkshire with her husband. She enjoys gardening, watching her husband bowling and researching.

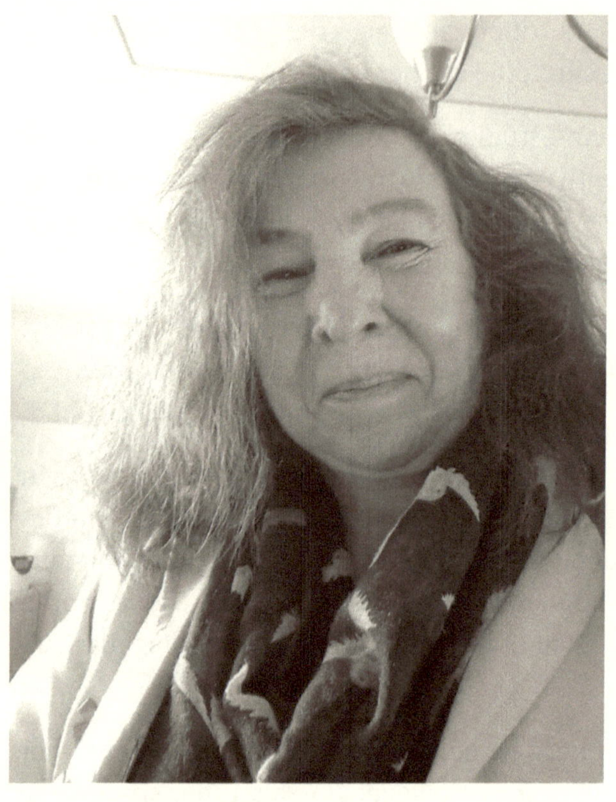

Author Lynne Noble at home

https://quintessentiallylynne.weebly.com/nutritional-medicine.html

Preface

When I began looking at the number of calorie restrictive diet books on the market, I was struck at how many removed essential food groups or withdrew - or severely restricted - the foods that they actually enjoyed. 'Going on a diet' appeared to be a form of self-flagellation – a punishment for being 'greedy' for eating more calories that we required. After all, we are told, 'all calories are the same.' But what if that is not true? Is it really that simple? What about those people who do diet, rigidly eating 'all the right things' but do not appear to lose an ounce? Is there a reason for that? Well yes, there is. Not all calories are equal but the calories in some types of chocolate are more equal than others.

It is quite possible to lose weight, quickly, healthily and without hunger on the chocolate diet. There is very sound scientific evidence for this which I will share with you in this book.

The chocolate diet is not suitable for everyone though. There are contraindications for those with:

- Alcoholism
- Cystic fibrosis

- Those individuals who have medical conditions relating to the thyroid
- Diabetes
- Angina
- Have had a heart attack
- High blood pressure
- Constipation – due to the high iron content in the chocolate, it can dysregulate the bowel
- Migraine – some migraineurs find that chocolate brings on a migraine attack fairly rapidly.
- This diet is not suitable for people with a viral infection.
- Those with a connective tissue disorder, as an ingredient in chocolate suppresses the COL 1 mRNA which codes for the protein collagen.

Nevertheless, weight loss can impact positively on some of these conditions so if you still want to go ahead then proceed with watchful caution. In the case of diabetics, the main consideration is that the chocolate should have no added sugar or have less than 2% of the recommended dietary allowance per two squares.

Fortunately, there is an abundance of no added sugar chocolate on the market at far less cost than many of the slimming products available on the market.

Does this diet work? Yes, I have personally tried it on myself after noticing that when I increased my chocolate intake – of a specific type – that I lost weight easily, happily and without hunger.

It seems to be too good to be true so maybe it is time to look at why not all calories are equal and why exercise does not work for all individuals embarking on a weight loss regime.

Adenosine

Not many people have heard of adenosine never mind know what it does. However, it is an important nutritional substance when it comes to understanding why weight loss may not occur - even after rigorous dieting.

 Adenosine is a regulatory molecule in metabolic processes. A metabolic process is a set of life supporting processes in an organism. They have one of three functions.

1. The conversion of food to energy so enable the basic functions of every cell.
2. The conversion of food to the basic building blocks for:

a) lipids which are fatty acids and glycerol.
b) protein which are amino acid
c) carbohydrates which are monosaccharides

d) nucleic acids which are nucleotides
3. The elimination of nitrogenous – or waste by-products –

Sometimes, the word metabolism refers to the total processes that allow the body to run efficiently.

Therefore, metabolic processes are vital for health.

In the brain, adenosine is a neurotransmitter (brain chemical that carries messages) that has an inhibitory action. It promotes sleep. Levels of adenosine rise throughout the day in response to exercise. This is an important concept that we shall return to shortly.

At the end of the day provided adenosine levels are high enough then arousal is suppressed and sleep promoted.

Adenosine has many other actions including energy metabolism and expenditure.

The more physical exercise that you do the more the more adenosine is produced. Adenosine helps muscles to adapt to exercise thus helping to prevent trauma. In addition, adenosine is also released in response to:

- Trauma of any kind
- Oxidative stress – where it helps to protect the brain
- Metabolic distress

Adenosine is found in all organs in the body where it has a diversity of functions including:

Kidneys – decreased blood flow and decreased production of rennin from the kidney.

Lungs – constriction of airways

Liver – constriction of blood vessels and increased breakdown of glycogen to form glucose

Heart – decreased heart rate and has antiplatelet action and increased diameter of blood vessels in peripheral organs.

Adenosine's numerous functions include:

- Relaxing vascular smooth muscle
- Regulating T cell proliferation and cytokine production - cytokines are small proteins that are secreted by cells of the immune system and have an effect on other cells.
- Relieving nerve pain including shingles
- **Inhibiting lipolysis**

Inhibiting lipolysis is the one that we are interested in. Lipolysis is the breakdown of fat. Fats are broken down in our body by enzymes and water. Fat is actually stored energy and found in adipose tissue stores. Fat has many uses including cushioning our bodies from trauma. Excess calories – over and above our needs – are stored as triglycerides and broken down when we need the energy that is stored there. This energy is useful in times of illness or when appetite is lost. The stored fat is broken down into fatty acids and glycerol providing an easily accessible form of fuel for the body. It effects this as adenosine is used in the composition of adenosine triphosphate, also known as ATP.

ATP provides energy which is required to fuel many of the processes in living cells. For example, you cannot contract muscles without it or initiate nerve impulses.

The importance of ATP is demonstrated by its description of

The molecular unit of currency of intracellular energy transfer

Now ATP is synthesised from fatty acids and protein from lean meats - chicken and turkey, for example, and also from fatty fish and nuts. However, as adenosine inhibits lipolysis, eating these foods – including chicken and turkey – have to potential to increase weight gain or the breakdown of fat for fuel. This may take some time to get your head around. We are so used to hearing that turkey and chicken are ideal foods for weight loss and in some respects – within a calorie controlled diet - they may be. However, we cannot look at any food in the light of how many calories a portion contains. Any food has numerous nutritional substances contained within it and each of those will interact with an individual's genetic makeup and impact on many aspects of overall health. Any of those other substances may promote or suppress weight gain. Currently, weight reducing diets have a tendency to restrict one of four factors:

- Carbohydrates
- Fat
- Protein
- Calories

However, there are many other nutrients in any food that may also have a bearing on an individual's body mass including adenosine. However, organisations or individuals, in the diet business, will address the factor that is the simplest one to address and further, will also maximise profits at the same time.

We also note that, as adenosine levels rise in response to exercise, then the breakdown for fat as a fuel is inhibited. This offers an explanation why exercise does not appear to be a good weight loss solution.   Indeed, for many – including me – exercising actually appears to increase weight gain. Some of this may be due to increased appetite but, in the majority, it cannot be explained by this

As adenosine containing foods are essential for energy transfer then we should not seek to limit them from our diet. However, we need to be aware that too many may – in genetically susceptible people – carry the risk for unwanted weight gain which is difficult to lose. Reducing the amount of foods containing adenosine during calorie restriction would aid the breakdown of stored fat.

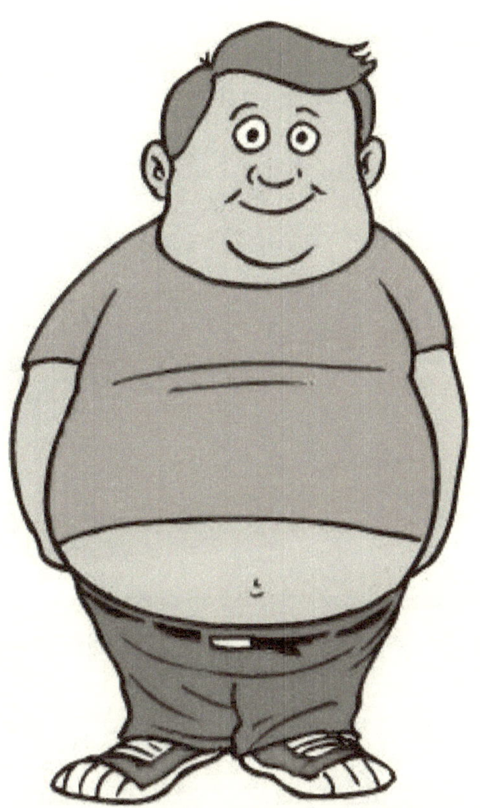

reducing foods containing adenosine would enable the breakdown of stored fat for energy.

I know of many individuals who embark on a diet and find that they are utterly exhausted and failing to lose weight. Many of the foods that are recommended for calorie restricted diets also contain the most amounts of adenosine.

---

[1] https://www.clipart.email/clipart/fat-people-clipart-3171.html

Therefore, the energy stored as triglycerides in fat cells, is not available to be used.

What are the main food sources of adenosine?

Adenosine is found in lean meats such as turkey and chicken, oily fish and nuts.

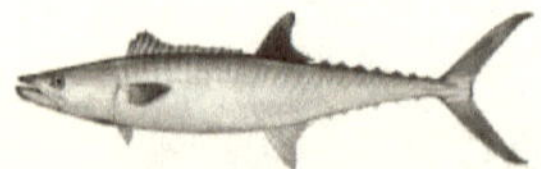

Mackerel contains good amounts of adenosine and therefore inhibits the breakdown of stored fat into a form that can be used.

However, we should not seek to exclude these foods from our diet as they contain many valuable nutrients. We merely need to reduce the amount of adenosine, in our diet, if our intake is high, or at least block some of the adenosine from being taken up by the body.

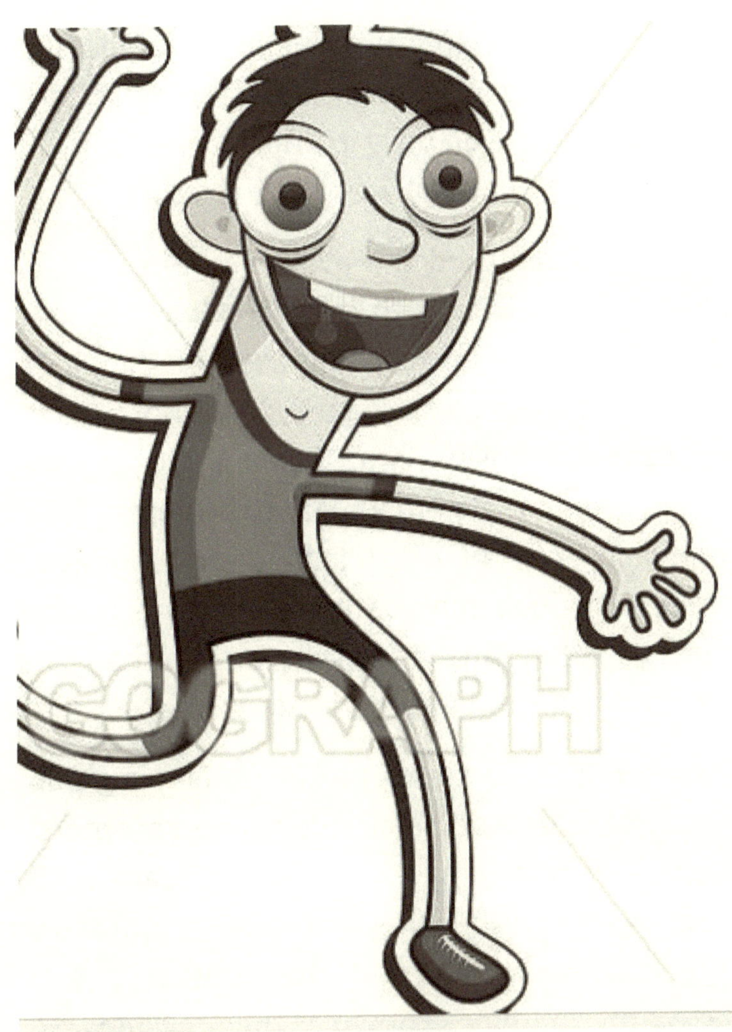

[2]Running increases the amount of adenosine in the body and inhibits the breakdown of fat.

---

[2] gg56845818

It can be understood from the above that dietary recommendations which include lean meat, oily fish and exercise, actually inhibit lipolysis. In fact, it flies in the face of all we have been told.

When we have used the available glucose, our hope is that calorie restriction and exercise will result in our fat stores being used for fuel and resulting in weight loss. Clearly, this is not always the case. Adenosine is an explanation of why some individuals do not appear to be able to lose weight in spite of disciplined dieting. Indeed, some individuals may be more sensitive to the effects of adenosine in their diet. What then can we do to block the effects of adenosine?

The answer lies in the methylxanthines – a group of substances that block adenosine receptors. Most people have never heard of methylxanthines but they will have undoubtedly eaten a common food stuff that contains one of the methylxanthines known as theophylline.

It is to the subject of theophylline that we now turn.

The Methylxanthines

Theophylline is a drug that is often used to treat respiratory disorders such as asthma and chronic obstructive pulmonary disease. It helps to relax bronchioles enabling easier airflow through the respiratory tract. It is also anti-inflammatory in action. However, for the purposes of the subject of this book, it is also an adenosine antagonist. What exactly is meant by that?

On every cell there will be tiny receptors for adenosine. These receptors are specifically shaped to grab hold of adenosine and no other substance. Sometimes, though, there are substances that can interfere or inhibit the functioning of another. Theophylline interferes with the action of adenosine preventing its ability to inhibit the breakdown of fat into useable fuel for the body. As one of adenosine's functions is to induce sleep, increasing theophylline in large amounts can cause insomnia.

Theophylline is found in tea (camellia sinensis) However, it is doubtful whether a nightly cup of tea contains enough theophylline to keep anyone awake. However, the main source of theophylline is cocoa. Dark chocolate which contains cocoa solids of 85% or upwards contains useful amounts of theophylline which acts as an adenosine antagonist.

 Drinking cocoa or eating dark chocolate, high in cocoa solids, helps the breakdown of fat.

Theophylline is not the only methylxanthine. As all methylxanthines have a role as antagonist of the adenosine receptors A_1 and A_2 then it is helpful if we look at some other common ones.

Caffeine and theobromine are the most abundant naturally occurring of methylxanthines.

Theobromine – also found in cocoa – improves your circulation and respiratory system. It increases the activity of a cell called cyclic adenosine monophosphate (cAMP). This messenger molecule activates an enzyme which reduces inflammation.

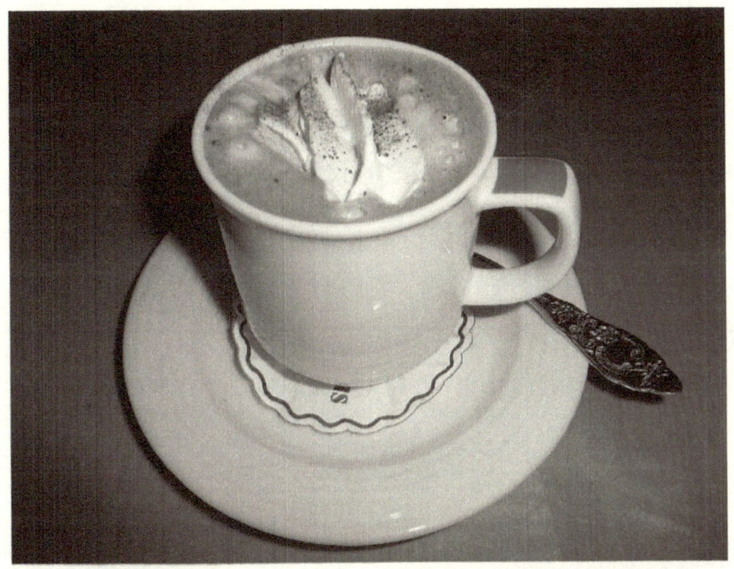

Cocoa can help with weight loss by the action of theophylline on adenosine receptors. A cup of cocoa contains approximately 170mg of theobromine.

The association of obesity with inflammation is now well established.

Given the impact of cocoa as a super food, why dark chocolate, with very high amounts of cocoa solids, is often limited - in weight loss diets – to a couple of squares is beyond me. It can be eaten in greater quantities and more often than is normally advised.

Caffeine is also a methylxanthine. It is the main methylxanthine of coffee where it has alerting effects. Its impact on the adenosine receptors is the reason why this stimulant keeps us awake if we drink it, in coffee, near bedtime.

On a personal level, I have found that when my intake of dark chocolate goes up replacing desserts – although the calories or more or less equal – I always lose significant amounts of weight during that period. This may be due to another of the methylxanthines considerable therapeutic effects- that of acting as a diuretic.

One of my acquaintances who had been dieting for some time expressed surprise that they had lost 3lb one week. When I asked why they were surprised the response was that they had been eating a lot of chocolate that week. It did not surprise me though.

This diuretic effect also has the ability to reduce blood pressure. It seems that the positive impact that chocolate - containing very high amounts of cocoa solids has - extends far beyond what we initially assumed we knew.

In addition, given chocolate's ability to open airways, we are more likely to want to exercise since we will suffer less breathlessness when doing so.

What does the chocolate diet look like then? Is it something that we can fit into our busy lives without too much thinking about?

The answer is yes. Chocolate is a superfood and deserves more of a place in our lives but I am not talking about milk chocolate or white chocolate. Milk chocolate contains very little of the methylxanthines while white chocolate contains none at all. When I refer to chocolate for the purposes of the chocolate diet referred to in this book I am referring to the dark chocolate containing at least 85% cocoa solids.

I will also be referring to cocoa. When I refer to cocoa most people think I mean drinking

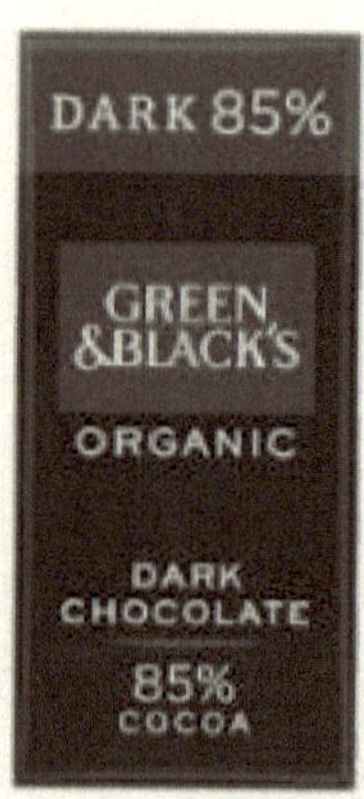

chocolate but drinking chocolate is not pure cocoa. Most of drinking chocolate is sugar and cannot be used for dietary purposes at all. When I refer to cocoa I mean just that, pure cocoa solids without any added sugar. Pure cocoa can be a little bitter so sweetener may be added to taste at any time.

Now that we have established what our sources of methylxanthines are to be, it is quite likely you want to quickly discover how quickly – and well -

the chocolate diet can fit into a daily regime. However, we need to look at some further amazing properties that the chocolate diet can bring. To this end we will look at chocolate as a polyphenol in our weight management programme. However, it may be useful to look at the diversity of nutrients that high quality chocolate contains.

In a 100g bar of chocolate there can be found

- 60% of the recommended daily intake (RDI) of iron (please note that iron cannot be absorbed without the addition of vitamin C).
- Over half of the RDI of magnesium
- 89% of copper (copper is an excellent antibacterial)
- Nearly the full RDI for manganese
- 11g of fibre (please note though that due to the high iron content of chocolate, it can be constipating)
- The fats are mostly saturated which means that they are stable and therefore do not cause inflammation. Chocolate

also contains some beneficial monounsaturated fats, too.

In addition, there are many other nutrients in lesser quantities. High quality chocolate is really a superfood.

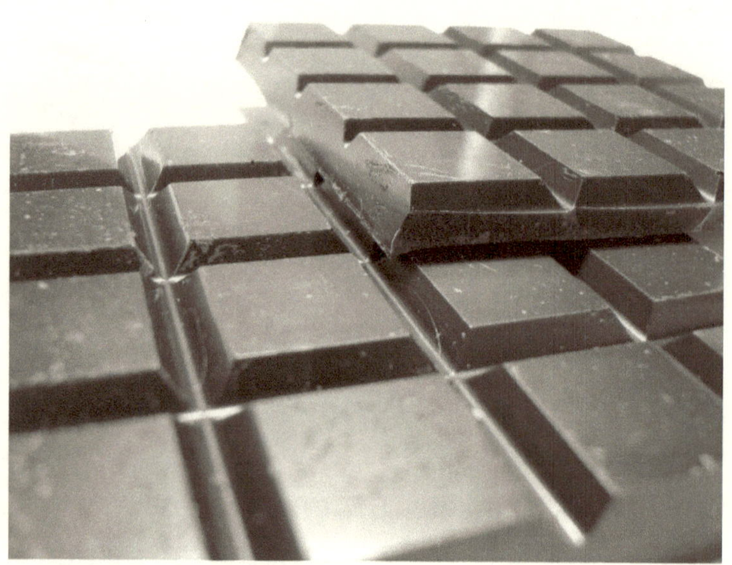

Chocolate as a Polyphenol

A Granada university study have scientifically disproved that eating chocolate is fattening. In an article published in the journal *Nutrition* it was reported that the higher the consumption of chocolate the less deposition of total fat throughout the body and the less central (abdominal) fat there was. This was regardless of whether the individual was dieting or engaged in exercise.

The body fat percentage was measured by skin folds and bioelectrical impedance analysis as well as waist circumference.

More recently, a cross sectional study in adults conducted by the University of California found that a lower body mass index was associated with more frequent chocolate consumption. There are good reasons for thinking this. Chocolate is a polyphenol. Polyphenols are micronutrients found in plant based foods. The specific polyphenol which has a therapeutic effect in chocolate is known as a catechin. Catechins are known to impact on cortisol production and on insulin sensitivity. When cortisol production is raised then fat stores are more easily laid down. Catechins can prevent this process. As such they can help with weight management although their mode of action on health extends far beyond that.

Other sources of catechins include tea and berries but by far the best source is cocoa and products made from it. It appears that dipping strawberries - or other berries - in chocolate, really has health giving properties.

Chocolate – the stimulant, antidepressant with antioxidant properties

Chocolate is both an antioxidant and also has stimulant and antidepressant properties. How do these characteristics help in a weight loss regime?

Studies have shown that individuals who are more depressed tend to eat more chocolate than those who did not suffer from this condition. Studies have shown that serotonin is increased when chocolate is eaten. The properties of serotonin are harnessed in antidepressants known as SSRI's. Serotonin is a neurotransmitter (brain chemical) that is released when we are in love. Serotonin also helps to control anxiety. Excessive eating and anxiety often go hand in hand so small amounts of chocolate can control binge eating.

Chocolate also contains small amounts of a compound called phenylethylamine. Phenylethylamine has an amphetamine type mode of action. It helps to release dopamine – another important neurotransmitter. Why is dopamine important? Most people will have heard of it in connection with Parkinson's disease but not actually know how it contributes to overall mental health.

Dopamine functions both as a hormone and a neurotransmitter. That is, it sends signals to other cells. Dopamine's strength lies in its ability to enhance reward motivated behaviour so that when we anticipate reward it will increase the level of dopamine in the brain. It enhances the states of happiness and a connection with others. It is not surprising that dopamine is known as the chemical of pleasure.

When looking at dopamine as a potential weight loss enhancer, it helps to know that depressive states inhibit norepinephrine. Dopamine can prevent this state. In addition, dopamine, as well as acting as a vasodilator in the kidney, increases sodium output. It also enhances urine flow. What is the significance of inhibiting norepinephrine?

When norepinephrine is inhibited then arousal and alertness is decreased. Reaction time is also reduced and concentration is also impacted. Many dieters will testify to the fact that they are unable to concentrate and lack motivation to follow calorie restriction through after a few days. Calorie restriction, after all, reduces the amount of food that contains dopamine and, I may add, the precursor to serotonin, so it is not surprising that it impacts on mood and motivation in this way. We cannot just restrict calories and believe that all will be plain sailing and that it cannot and will not impact on us during this time. It is bound to if we are not judicious in what we are doing.

Chocolate also has antioxidant properties. Exactly what do we mean by this?

Antioxidants help to prevent oxidation. Oxidation is a chemical reaction that can produce free radicals. Free radicals are unpaired electrons. When electrons are unpaired they are unstable. In the process of finding another electron to pair up with, they cause a lot of damage to other cells. The damage can manifest itself as changes seen in the ageing process. Free radical damage can result in illness such as cancers. It has also been linked to arthritis, stroke, heart disease, emphysema and other respiratory disorders. Parkinson's disease as well as countless other medical conditions where inflammation is known to play a part.

The antioxidant in cocoa has a particular structure that places it as a flavonoid. The three main flavonoids in cocoa are:

- Procyanidin
- Epicatechin
- Catechins

By far the greatest flavonoid antioxidant found in chocolate is procyanidin. Procyanidin has some excellent health enhancing properties.[3] It can:

- Inhibit oxidised Low Density Lipoprotein
- Improve glucose intolerance
- Scavenge free radicals very effectively

---

[3] https://www.ncbi.nlm.nih.gov/pmc/articles/PMC4696435/

- Directly influence insulin resistance and thus reduce risk for diabetes
- Protect nerves from injury and inflammation
- Protect skin from oxidative damage especially in relation to skin exposure

These beneficial effects are just the tip of the iceberg.

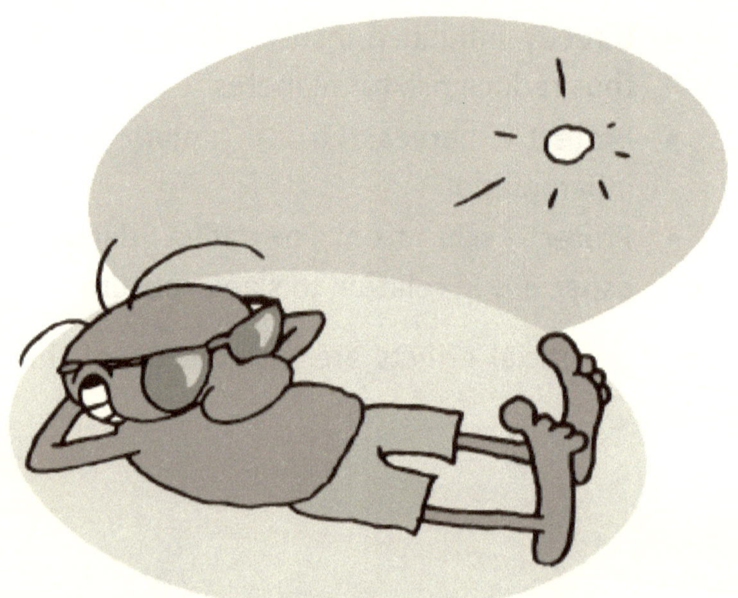

4 **cocoa can help protect your skin from oxidative damage**

After this brief, but valuable look, at the benefits of eating high cocoa solid chocolate perhaps we ought to now look at the chocolate diet and how it can be incorporated into your daily eating regime. So, it is to this that we will now turn.

---

4 http://clipart-library.com/tanning-people-cliparts.html

The Chocolate Diet

Before you embark on this diet you will need to take a few measurements and log them. Thereafter, you will need to log them on a weekly basis, preferably first thing in the morning. A log for this purpose is provided for you on the next page. You can either photocopy it or draw up your own up after the one below is used.

You will need to be prepared to buy at least one bar of 85% cocoa solids chocolate each day which is at least 90g. Most of the bars of dark chocolate come in 90g bars. I have also sourced dark chocolate which contains 90% cocoa solids but I imagine it would be very bitter and not to everyone's taste. The chocolate must not contain nuts nor any of the fruit flavoured bits that often accompany this type of chocolate.

You will also need to buy pure cocoa.

The diet can be adapted to suit your lifestyle – I will come back to that concept in a minute but, given that methylxanthines are stimulants and diuretics it is recommended that most of the chocolate and cocoa is taken early in the day. Theophylline does not have a long half-life but nevertheless, may disrupt some individuals sleep. You will find out how chocolate affects you and adapt your eating pattern to suit.

Exercise is important if for the only reason that it enables the flow of lymph. The lymphatic glands do not have an external pump in the way that the circulatory system has the heart as a pump. Gentle exercise is required to move lymph around the lymphatic system.

I am not advocating that you suddenly take up cross country running. A gentle stroll down to the shop or library is fine. As we have already discovered exercise can inhibit lipolysis.

Nevertheless, exercise is necessary to keep muscles and the lymphatic system functioning well.

The Log

Date		
weight	kg	lb
measurement	cm	Inches
Under bust or chest measurement		
Waist		
Hips		
Above knee		
Around wrist		

It should be made clear that the above measurements are the most useful ones but that should not stop you adding other if you desire. You may wish to provide a more bespoke log recording any pluses or minuses in the weekly measurements you make. For example, if you have thick ankles you may wish to measure and record ankle diameter, on a weekly basis, before you start this diet.

There are few rules. Two mugs of cocoa are to be drunk every day but the timing is to suit you although earlier in the day is probably best for most people. I can never understand why cocoa was marketed as a night cap when it has the capacity to cause insomnia.

A 90g bar of chocolate as previously outlined must be eaten every day. Two squares should be eaten at least half an hour before a meal but the rest may be eaten when you desire. In addition, another two squares should be eaten before you set out on your daily exercise regime – walking to the bus stops or local shops

In addition, you may use another 45g of chocolate from a second bar in desserts or as extra snacks throughout the day. One of my friends melts it and swirls it over a banana. The possibilities for using chocolate are limited only by the imagination.

That's it really. It is that simple.

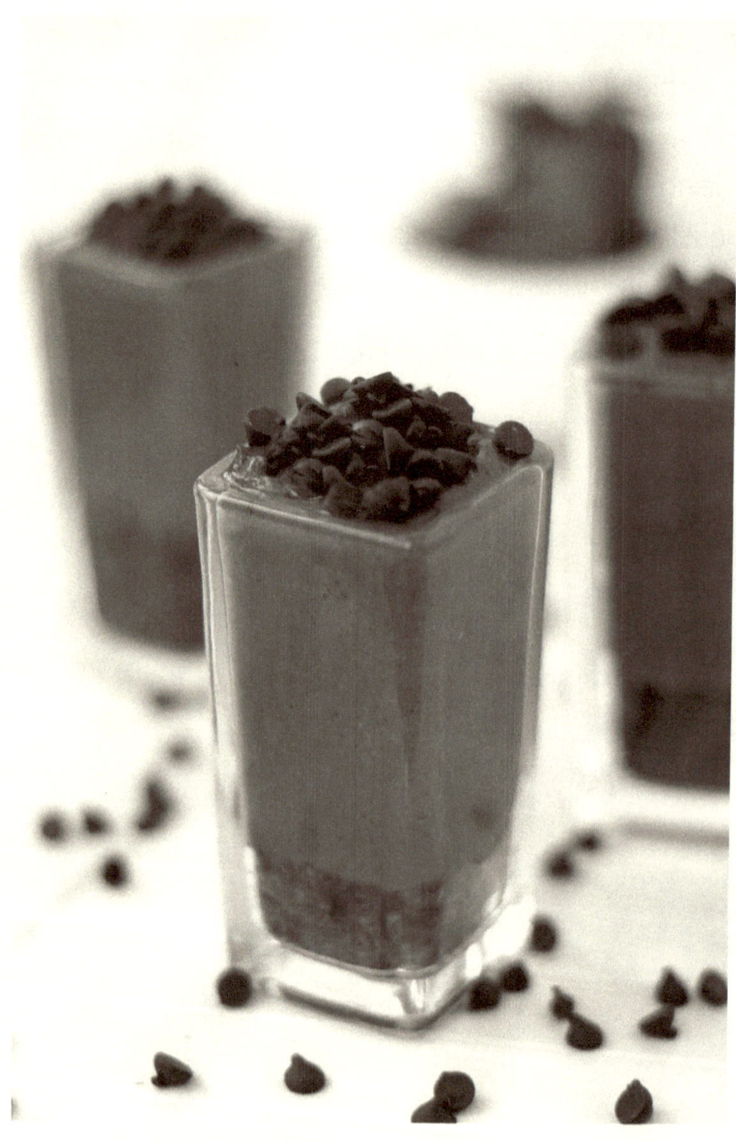

The use of chocolate is limited only by the imagination.

One of the easiest chocolate desserts that you can make consists of three ingredients

- 85% melted cocoa solid chocolate
- Quark
- Sweetener

They need to be whisked together and allowed to set. Of course, you can add bits of zest from orange peel or a sprig of mint or maybe just a pinch of cinnamon. Whatever you choose to do the chocolate diet is full of health giving nutritional substances, is tasty and is not so complicated, or restrictive, that the dieter is likely to give up on it after a week.

It is also certainly cheaper than many calorie-counted dieting meals, does not need preparation, or cooking, and can be carried everywhere with you.

The beauty is in its simplicity.

Other benefits of the chocolate diet

High cocoa solid chocolate contains excellent amounts of copper. In fact, three ounces of dark 85% cocoa solid chocolate contains slightly more than the recommended daily intake of copper.

The significance of this is more profound at this current time. As I write the Coronavirus pandemic has reached sensationalist proportions in the media with wildly diverse predictions of what may happen if people do not self-isolate from those who may potentially be harbouring the virus.

Most of the panic seems to be driven by reports that this is a de novo virus which the immune system has not come across before. In truth, any infection which manifests itself in any individual is one that the immune system has not come across before. However, the immune system is able to respond to any de novo infection that arises provided that all the correct nutrients required to make immune system cells and innate defences are present.

The Coronavirus is reported to be more likely to produce severe symptoms, or death, in older people and those with underlying medical conditions. There is good reason for this.

Elderly people tend to have depleted levels of a number of nutrients that are essential for the smooth running of the immune system. There are a number of reasons for this including a poor diet, poor appetite and an inability to absorb any nutrients ingested as well as they were able, when younger.

Copper has excellent antiviral and antibacterial properties. Infective agents are killed on contact with copper. Research from the University of Southampton[5] has found that copper can effectively help to prevent the spread of respiratory viruses including animal coronaviruses. When viruses came into contact

---

[5] https://www.sciencedaily.com/releases/2015/11/151110102147.htm

with copper the viral genome and the structure of viral particles were destroyed. This included those of influenza A.

Copper is able to:

- Prevent cell respiration
- Destroy DNA and RNA thus preventing the virus from mutating
- Punches holes in bacterial cells membranes
- Disrupts the viral coat

Copper's diverse effects respond to the two main stages found in the Coronavirus strategy.

The virus may kill in younger people, mainly, due to the destruction of tissue by the host as it battles infection by a virus. The immune system has a tendency to go overboard in young people whereas in children and the elderly, the immune system is likely to respond more sedately.

The immune system's response includes the proliferation of white blood cells, antibodies and inflammatory mediators. T cells destroy any tissue harbouring any virus but they can go 'over the top' as they do in autoimmune diseases and destroy too much lung tissue.

More virulent strains trigger a stronger inflammatory response but having enough copper in the diet can respond to viral infection before it can take hold.

The destruction of respiratory tissue is not what has allegedly caused the death of elderly. This appears to have been due to secondary pneumonia. Pneumonia can be either viral or bacterial in origin. However, as those with Coronavirus induced pneumonia are given antibiotics we must assume that it is caused by a bacterial infection of *streptococcus or staphylococcus origin.* Pneumonias caused by these can cause septic shock and multiple organ failure.

Some pneumonias are viral in origin but copper can respond to both viral and bacterial pneumonias as well as the initial stages of infection by the virus.

Thus, cocoa and dark chocolate, high in cocoa solids, are an effective weapon in the battle against infections caused by viral and bacterial infections. In addition, chocolate has been found to have anti-fungal properties, too.

Zinc has potent antiviral properties and many people take zinc at the first sign of infection. However, copper and zinc compete for absorption. Therefore, if you do take zinc at the first sign of infection, then foods containing high amounts of copper should be taken some hours apart.

Foods containing high amounts of copper beside chocolate are:

- Brazil nuts
- Trout
- Liver
- Peanut butter
- Seeds
- avocado

Chocolate recipes

This one is so easy to make and takes only minutes to do. My favourite recipe by far.

Ingredients

- Melted chocolate 85% cocoa solids or above
- Chopped dried fruit
- Coarsely chopped digestive biscuits
- Desiccated coconut

Additional extra – small petit four cases

Melt enough chocolate so that it binds the other ingredients – dried fruit and biscuit - together.

Roll into small balls about 2.5cm in diameter. When nearly set, roll in the desiccated coconut and place in the petit four cases

Alternative version

Try chopped glace cherry and chopped almonds with the melted chocolate.

Chocolate custard

This is such an easy recipe to make. I generally make a chocolate sponge and microwave it to go with this.

Ingredients

- one rounded dessertspoon of cocoa powder
- cornflour to thicken about one dessertspoon
- sweetener to taste
- Two dessertspoons of skimmed milk powder

Method

Place all the ingredients in a microwaveable jug. Add a little cold water until all mixed together well.

Add 15 fluid ounces of boiling water stirring all the time. You may need to use a hand whisk to get a really smooth custard

If it hasn't thickened properly then place in the microwave for ten seconds at a time, observing closely for thickening. Take out and whisk again for a really smooth sauce.

Sometimes, I add broken pieces of dark chocolate to the sauce to give it an extra boost.

Ingredients (four people)

- Two large eggs
- Four ounces of self-raising flour
- Sweetener
- One heaped dessertspoon of cocoa

- Two ounces of butter

Method

Add all ingredients together and mix well.

Place in a microwaveable basin.

Microwave for four minutes. Test to see if it is set by inserting a knife to see if it comes out clean. The sponge will be very hot so caution is needed.

If the sponge is not set, then microwave for another 30 seconds and another 30 seconds thereafter. Leave to stand for one minute before serving.

Small squares of chocolate can be inserted into the sponge before it is left to rest. This will add a little extra decadence to your dessert.

Variations

Various flours can be substituted for the self-raising flour including soya flour. If non self-raising flours are used, then you will need to add some bicarbonate of soda to enable the mixture to rise. In addition, ground almonds can be substituted for part of the flour. This adds a richer flavour than using wheat flour alone.

Using different flours other than wheat flour may take a little trial and error to find the correct blend of flour and/or added ground almonds and a raising agent.

As an easy and tasty hot dessert I don't mind if the shape is not perfect. It is the taste that counts for me.

To counteract any tendency to dryness, I sometimes add a little coconut oil or use desiccated coconut to add a little moistness to the mix.

Eggs can be replaced with pureed apple. The apple binds the mixture in the way that eggs do. The texture of the sponge is different but still delightful.

Bananas can also be mashed into the flour mix. Chocolate and banana go together well.

Baked chocolate egg custard

Ingredients

- 300mls full fat milk
- 200 mls of pouring cream
- 100g of 85% cocoa solid chocolate
- 4 egg yolks
- 50 – 100 of sweetener to taste
- 1 teaspoon of vanilla extract

Method

Preheat oven to 150C

Add milk and cream together into a saucepan. Stir until just at the point of simmer.

Remove the pan from the heat.

Add the chocolate and allow it to melt into the liquid. Stir until smooth.

Whisk the egg yolks, vanilla essence and sugar in a heat proof bowl.

Pour the hot milk over this and whisk until very smooth.

Place this mixture into individual ramekin dishes or a dish for a non-individual custard.

Place on a baking tray and pour boiling water into the baking tray until it comes up to the side of the dishes containing the egg custard

Bake for about 45 minutes – longer if it is one larger dish – until it is just set.

To microwave, cook on 50% power for 4 minutes, leave for 30 seconds to see if the egg custard has set.

Variations

If you wish to add cocoa instead of the chocolate pieces, then this also works well. The cocoa needs a good whisk in to the warm milk as it tends to form clumps easily.

Whatever you use it is important to test the mixture for sweetness – not everyone likes the slight bitterness that dark chocolate imparts.

Chocolate Soup – pure decadence

Ingredients (serves 4 small portions)

- 200ml of double cream
- 200g of 85% pure cocoa solid chocolate
- 100ml of strong coffee
- 5 tbsp of brandy

Method

Place the cream in a saucepan over a gentle heat and bring to the boil.
Prepare the coffee.
Throw in pieces of chocolate to the warmed cream. Once blended and smooth add the coffee and brandy.

Serve in individual dishes and add vanilla ice cream if desired.

85% Chocolate Brownies (recipe provided by Rob Williams, with thanks).

Serves 9 Preparation: 10 minutes

Ingredients:

4 oz of 85% dark chocolate broken into small pieces

8tbsp of unsalted melted butter

1 cup of castor sugar

¼ tsp vanilla extract

¼ tsp salt

2/3 eggs depending on size

1/3 cup of plain flour

Method:

Heat the oven to 180C/350f/gas mark 4

Prepare an 8 inch square pan by lining it with parchment paper

In a microwaveable bowl, microwave the chocolate on half power in 30 second bursts, stirring in between until the chocolate is melted and smooth and then set aside to cool until just warm.

In a large bowl whisk together the melted butter, sugar, vanilla and salt and then whisk in the eggs one at a time

Stir in the cooled melted chocolate into the ingredients mixed and add in the flour until combined.

Once mixed, scrape the batter into the prepared pan and bake for 20-30 minutes in the middle of the oven. Test the bake, after the cooking time, with a knife to see if it comes out clean. This indicates that the brownie is cooked.

Place the pan on a rack for 10-20 minutes to allow the brownie to cool and then remove the brownie completely from the pan to allow it to cool further.

Serving suggestions:

Serve with clotted cream or ice cream with grated orange rind on the top.

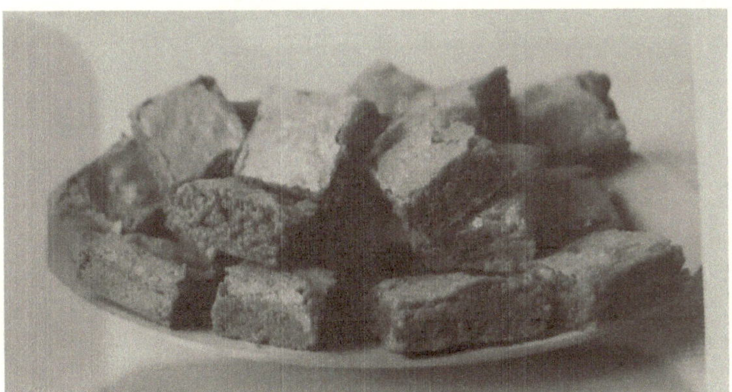

Braised Beef with Chilli and Chocolate Recipe (with thanks to Rob Williams for contributing this recipe)

Serves 6   Preparation: 5-10 minutes Cooking time: 2 1/2 hours-3 hours

Ingredients:

2 tbsp vegetable oil

Pinch of salt

Pinch of pepper

1 heaped tbsp. of plain flour

3 lbs of diced stewing beef

3 large carrots roughly chopped

1 onion roughly chopped

1 tbsp of cumin seeds

1 tbsp of ground coriander

Large pinch of chilli powder

Small stick of cinnamon

1 whole red chilli

Half a pint of red wine or porter beer

12 oz of beef stock

14 oz of chopped tomatoes (two tins)

Large thyme sprig

2 bay leaves

2 oz of 85% dark chocolate.

Method:

Heat the oven to 180C/gas mark 4/ 160f fan

Heat the oil in a large flame proof casserole dish

Add the salt and pepper to the flour and coat the beef with it

Brown the coated beef in the heated oil in batches and cook

Add in the vegetables to the same pot as the beef and brown slightly

Stir in the spices and add the chill and then cook further for a few minutes

Pour in the wine, stock and chopped tomatoes to the dish

Add the herbs and bring to a simmer

Once simmering. Cover with a lid and put in the oven for an hour and a half

After this time, remove the lid and cook for a further hour or until the meat is tender

When cooked, remove from the oven and leave to cool slightly

Finally stir in the chocolate and serve

Serving suggestion:

Plate up with mash or boiled potatoes or for a different variation, rice.

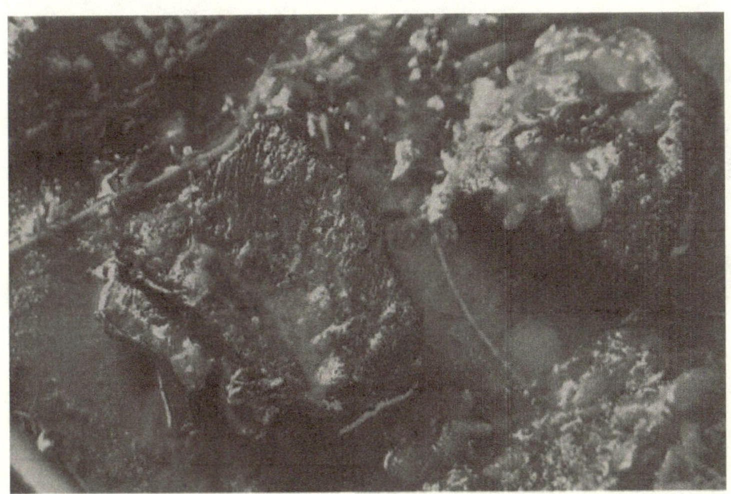

Braised beef with chilli and chocolate

Information for diabetics

At the beginning of this book I did warn that this diet may not be suitable for diabetics even though weight loss is desirable for those with diabetes type 2. There are a number of reasons why this should be but the primary one is that the chocolate diet can increase insulin sensitivity and decrease blood pressure. Unless a diabetic is vigilant in monitoring changes on a daily basis then problems may arise.

Insulin sensitivity simply refers to how sensitive the body's cells are in response to insulin. High insulin sensitivity means that the cells in the body can use glucose in an efficient way. This means that there is less circulating blood sugar.

Low circulating blood sugar is desirable because when blood sugar levels are high then it has the potential to increase the risk of infection, contributes to poor wound healing, tiredness, brain fog (since the cells are now powered by glucose) damage to nerves, known as neuropathy - which includes damage to the kidneys and eyes - and an increased risk of atherosclerosis which is a risk factor for heart disease and stroke.

Increasing insulin sensitivity sounds just the ticket but if the diabetic is insulin dependent and does not monitor their condition they may inject too much insulin and cause a hypoglycaemic attack where the blood sugar levels are too low.

The other factor that we need to monitor is that of blood pressure. Normally the blood pressure of diabetics is too high for comfort increasing the risk of cardiovascular events or stroke. Hypertension may be due to obesity or the narrowing of arteries due to atherosclerosis or both. There may be other factors at play but the high cocoa content of chocolate reduces abdominal fat and helps reduce the blood pressure.

Normally, diabetics are on a range of medications one of which reduces blood pressure. If this is not monitored when on the chocolate diet, then the blood pressure may drop too low. Very low blood pressure also carries with it, its own problems. It increases the likelihood of depression or low mood and fatigue. During the chocolate diet, the expectation is that blood pressure will drop and medication may need reducing. Therefore, unless the diabetic is vigilant in monitoring their blood sugar levels – and responding accordingly – and their blood pressure, this diet is not for them.

A percentage of the royalties from the sale of these books are used for charitable purposes. One such charity that has benefitted is the Exodus Project.

The Exodus Project

My first introduction to the far reaching impact of The Exodus Project occurred when I was travelling around Cawthorne in one of their buses, visiting gardens. A young lad was happily munching on a sandwich. He looked up briefly, pointed to the driver and said,' He's my second dad, he is,' then he returned to his sandwich without further comment

Such remarks are often very telling and so I arranged to meet Jackie Peel and Martin Sawdon, at the charity's premises in Barnsley. They set up the Exodus Project 20 years ago. They moved into their current premises – a redundant Methodist church - in 2010.

Both Jackie and Martin have been youth workers in their church. Martin worked in housing for the homeless in addition to working in learning disabilities services in institutional settings.

The work that the Exodus Project undertakes is of paramount importance to the communities it serves. These were former mining communities which became disadvantaged after pit-closures. Currently about 400 children attend mid-week activities from Monday to Thursday inclusive. These activities include dance, drama, craft, music, sports and games. In addition, there are weekend camps, cycle treks, outward bound activities, bowling and swimming. The children are taught valuable life skills including how to cook and bake. It is all about teaching children how to fulfil their potential and learn skills they will be able to pass onto the next generation.

The grounds, once overgrown, have been turned into a play- and camping - ground. A miniature railway is in the process of being installed.

Martin and Jackie have developed a unique model in that The Exodus Project goes beyond dispensing services. They are keen   to build up relationships with the whole family and not just the child that attends the mid- week clubs. In addition, once children have reached the age of fourteen, they are invited to help out with the younger groups as junior volunteers. Once they reach the age of eighteen, they become adult volunteers. This   model provides a constant supply of help from individuals who have benefitted already from attending such groups.

The   building is large and inviting. It is decorated with bold colours and has comfy seating. It is a real home from home; a haven for families who have been disadvantaged by the closure of the life force of its community.

Martin and Jackie have clear ideas about how they wish to develop the Exodus Project but the lottery funding which they benefitted from is no longer available. Sadly, they have had to close two of their clubs due to lack of funding. This decision   wasn't taken lightly. They do have two charity shops which raises some money and they obtain some funding from outside organisations for the use of their facilities. However, this is clearly not enough to keep their clubs, weekend activities   and building going to cater for the ever growing number of children who are benefitting from the work being undertaken here.   Neither does it allow for future development.

Exodus do have a Just Giving page which can be found here if you wish to help further their work https://www.justgiving.com/exodus

In addition, you can keep up with activities on their Facebook page here

https://www.facebook.com/search/top/?q=the%20exodus%20project%20barnsley&epa=SEARCH_BOX

If anyone wishes undertake an event like The Three Peaks - or run a marathon to raise funds for   Exodus - then Martin or Jackie would be pleased to hear from you. This will enable their vital work in the community to continue. Contact them through their website to be found on www.exodusproject.org.uk.